BUILDING A ROBUST IMMUNE SYSTEM

From Emotions to Pandemics

BY: AADIL A. ABBASI

ISBN: 9798664994643

Table of Contents

PREFACE

In today's world of inventions, even bacteria and viruses are not behind! Every day we hear about new diseases or germs affecting populations and communities. Have these germs advanced, or have human beings lost the tendency to cope with them? In this book, I have tried to cover all the questions that may help you to discover how you can prepare your body to overcome the presently functional pathogens worldwide or yet new to appear. Who knows?

Our immune systems play a vital role in protecting our bodies against any foreign element that may try to attack. To help keep yourself completely armored, educating yourself with how "Building a Stronger Immune System" is essential. I have always been motivated to keep myself fit and healthy for my family. But my last visit to a hospital to see one of my friends, and knowing the number of patients increasingly growing encouraged to put down the importance of immunity on human health.

Saying this, the only solution we can think of surviving a pandemic is to implement the precautionary measures applied to it and taking care of our immune system. Our immune system would work for the defense of our bodies, creating a memory to fight against the germs and protecting us in the future too. Studies show that the majority of the death rates during a pandemic are within people with a weak immune system. Mostly very young and older people are vulnerable to infectious diseases because young are naive immunologically and due to undergoing immune senescence in older adults.

I have set all the efforts to collect intricate information on various aspects, including food, exercise, vitamins, emotions, hydration, weight loss, age, and sleep, that may help you in strengthening your immunity. While working with boosting immunity, you should not overdo it. Where it is crucial to work on a healthy immune system, it is also essential to retain the balance. Strong immunity means a sharp mind, body, and soul. Let us see in detail how it works and why it is essential.

Aadil A. Abbasi - https://healthyfitcare.com

01 July 2020

CHAPTER ONE

IMMUNE SYSTEM OVERVIEW

There is a whole empire of barbaric creatures residing in all of us. This empire is named the immune system. It has a collection of special machinery (organs), chemicals, and soldiers (cells) that fight against traitors (cancerous cells) and raiders called microbes who try to invade this land called Human Body. The immune system mainly consists of antibodies, white blood cells, the lymphatic system, the complement, the thymus, the spleen, and also the bone marrow. These parts of the immune system work actively to fight against infections.

Our immune system has a blessed memory and keeps a record of every microbe it may have ever defeated. Yes, the same way you remember your childhood victories! These are also known as memory cells, which are a type of white blood cell comprising of B- and T- lymphocytes. If any microbes attack your body, it recognizes it, opens up its defensive gadgets, attacks and destroys it before it may multiply in your body and make you ill.

Occasionally for some infections, during this action combat you can feel a rise in body temperature or fever, and this is a response from the immune system to kill some microbes. Fevers help to expedite the repairing process of the body.

It is essential to have a properly functioning and a robust immune system to move in with daily life as you contact thousands of germs and infections from other people, pets, and also your environment. Without having a robust immune system, you can easily pick diseases, especially infectious diseases that could beget severe effects on your health, whereas pandemics may also prove fatal.

In addition to microbes, our immune system also down-regulates immune responses, therefore, preventing the consequence of autoimmune diseases or allergies. Scientists have now researched the activation of immune cells that are blocked by Tregs (the regulatory T cells), which are part of the immune system.

We usually take our immune system for granted as it secretly functions around the clock for our defense and fighting infections that we don't even notice it. It is relatively significant to look after your immune system to make it more robust so that it can look after you better.

Working of Immune System

To understand in-depth about the immune system and how to boost it, you need to know what it is composed of. The immune system is mainly made up of white blood cells or leukocytes. These are originated from bone marrow. From there, they enter the bloodstream and the lymphatic system (A passageway that gets rids of toxins and other harmful substances). One released leukocyte watch for any suspicious substance in our body. White blood cells mainly rely on antigens, which are present in all living cells. These are traces that help us recognize a cell. Every human has it's on antigen type, and it doesn't accept anything other than its own antigen. White blood cells trace out the different antigens and attack accordingly.

Threats to our body are incredibly variable, and we encounter each challenge we have an assortment of white blood cells. The variety helps us to tackle different problems in unique ways. Despite this massive diversity of white blood cells, we mainly classify them as two major cellular groups—phagocytes and lymphocytes, which both of these two-pronged coordinate attacks.

Phagocytes include:

- Neutrophils — these are the most prevalent form of phagocyte which prefer to target bacteria.

- Monocytes — these are the essential type and have several roles.

- Macrophages — patrol these for pathogens and remove dead and dying cells as well.

- Mast cells — they have many jobs, including helping heal wounds and defending against pathogenic diseases.

Lymphocytes include:

- B lymphocytes — they generate antibodies and help notify T cells.

- T lymphocytes — they destroy the body's compromised cells and help warn other leukocytes.

- Helper T Cells – they help B lymphocytes to generate complex antibodies, mostly for novel antigens.

Firstly phagocyte finds the microbe and devours it all the types of phagocytes have the same function to locate and consume the bacterium. It is a crucial step because then phagocytes identify the microbe, which then sends the signal to the second major cell group, lymphocytes. Once they got the signal, T-cells rushes to the site of the emergency and starts fighting off harmful antigens. Meanwhile, B-cells and helper T-cells are making antibodies (which are proteins and enzymes), which helps get rid of the threat entirely and gives immunity for some time for that disease.

Can we really" boost" our immune system?

Our immune system is a natural body process, and this gives rise to this question if we can boost our immune system? It is just like asking if we can boost our circulatory, respiratory, or excretory system. The simple answer to this is NO. Ingrained immunity cannot be boosted, and you don't even want it to stimulate a well operational natural process.

You may have come across many products that insist on boosting your immunity, and it doesn't even make much sense scientifically. In general, as discussed above, our immune system consists of many different types of cells that are responsive to different kinds of microbes in particular ways. Which cell would you choose to boost, and to what extent? It is controversial scientifically.

However, researchers do confirm that our body makes immune cells, which are our white blood cells, also known as leukocytes. These leukocytes combine into an adaptive system consisting of B and T cells that get mature and are produced more than required, called the lymphocytes.

These extra cells then start destroying themselves through a natural process of cell death called apoptosis. This cell death plays an integral part in all aspects of an immune system to function. In response to pathogens, apoptosis allows the immune system and tends to turn it off. If our body detects a microbe, the immune cells that recognize it start dividing extensively, which, as a result of cell death or apoptosis, also kills the invader.

If our bodies somehow fail to undergo apoptosis, this causes some severe consequences directing to autoimmune diseases and malignant growth. These are conditions of a weak immune system or immunocompromised that may be a result of medications like corticosteroids or genetics. Remember that our immune system is not a single being; it is a military of the whole army. We can, however, work to strengthen our immune system overall by adopting a healthy lifestyle and a balanced strategy that may work in harmony with the system as a whole. Many factors can be linked to help in strengthening the system, thus making you less prone to infections and pandemics.

ARE VACCINATIONS IMPORTANT?

Vaccinations, also known as immunizations, are given to boost the ability of the immune system to fight against certain infections. It works by teaching your body's immune system to identify microbes or germ cells so that when they are exposed to them, they recognize them and kill them without making you sick. Hence, creating a defensive mechanism against any antibodies.

Infants are usually vaccinated in the first twelve months of their birth to make their immune system prepared for any antigen that they may be at risk as they grow up. Vaccinations are specific for certain diseases. These are the weak germ of illness to build the memory of the immune system to fight against antibodies. An injection usually injects vaccinations in the thigh or upper arm. Vaccines prevent bodies from many contagious diseases like influenza, measles, chickenpox, whooping cough, and so forth. If not controlled, these illnesses can also prove fatal.

Vaccinations are proved to protect forthcoming generations. The diseases that have killed or severely attacked previous generations have been reduced or even eliminated. One of the examples of it is smallpox that has been eradicated worldwide. We don't also need to have its vaccination now because the disease no longer exists. Another example of rubella (German measles), if injected to children, the risk that women giving birth to babies will pass the virus to the new-borns have drastically reduced. If we follow the vaccination procedures correctly and completed today, it is evident that some or most of the diseases that attack today would no longer exist in future generations.

Vaccination would always play a role in polymorphic health concerns of the public with the emergence of a pandemic disease. Where other measures are taken to control a pandemic such as treatments, personal precautionary equipment, quarantine, surveillance, deployment of vaccine is indispensable for protection and limit the spread of the virus. It is, however, disquieting to know that not all disease threats have affiliated vaccines, and for some, if they do have, they might not be safe to use during a pandemic and can face various challenges.

HISTORY OF IMMUNE SYSTEM.

An immune system is a unique software in our body that can learn and adapt to the changes in our collection. Our immune system was not this strong from the very beginning; little by little, we, with the help of our immune system, learned to live in the wilds. Which comes with deathly diseases that destroy millions of people. To prevent these diseases from spreading, our immune system encoded the data in our ancestor's DNA (Deoxyribonucleic Acid), which helps us to survive from the deadliest diseases of the past. Many pandemics destroyed the population of the world; the first plague ever recorded was Antonine Plague, which is believed to either measles or smallpox. It killed 5 Million people; at that time, it is 5% of the population. But eventually, this virus stopped spreading because our body got immune to it. It wasn't harmful anymore.

But four hundred years after humankind was inflicted with another plague names as Plague of Justinian, it started in 541 to 542, and in just two years, it killed 30-50 Million people, which is bizarre. Rats and fleas caused this pandemic. But the human race survived through it and started living with no problems. Our immune system now knows how to defeat that disease, and so it wasn't a threat anymore. Then out of nowhere, in Europe, seven hundred years after humanity experienced another wave of terrific monsters named Yersinia pestis bacterium in 1347. It took away two hundred million lives but luckily stopped in 1351.

After this, another wave of smallpox appeared in 1520, and this was way advanced than the first one in 541. It was mutated, and there was no other way to stop it. Luckily it wasn't as contagious as the first one, and the person who survives it creates immunity from it. Which is passed on centuries after centuries to next-generation that now smallpox is very rare to see. You probably never heard of it.

It means that our immune system grows with the environment around it to survive. Viruses and bacteria also get stronger over time that it becomes a threat to human existence. Simple flu caused by the Influenza virus in 1918 destroyed the world. It killed 50 million people, which is disastrous. But the human body becomes resilient to it, and the death toll started to come down year after year. But, flu remains in our society because it changes form every year and attacks us. Luckily our immune system is resilient enough to fight it back.

All these pandemics are the ones which we recovered from on our own or with just medicines and a little bit of help from our immune system. But there are some plagues from which our immune system is clueless. To fight these deadly monsters invading our bodies, we have to train our immune system. We can qualify our immune system through vaccines and other activities.

CHAPTER 2

DIET AND IMMUNE SYSTEM

There is no distinct food that will help in upgradations of your immune system. However, a poor diet can have adverse effects on the immune system. A properly balanced diet comprising of fruits and vegetables rich in vitamins and minerals is crucial for all body operations, including the immune system to function at its best. An excellent operating immune system needs further energy supply during infection attacks due to tremendous energy requirements same for instance, during a fever.

This demand for nutrition and energy for the immune system to operate functionally is fulfilled only by the external source of food. Decent energy supply allows the immune system to initiate a response to infections, besides, to resolve an attack whenever needed and to avoid any elementary chronic inflammation.

Some dietary elements play a significant role in the maintenance and development of a well-operated immune system for a lifetime. For instance, amino acid arginine and micronutrients like Vitamin A and Zinc assist cell division and are proved to be successful in the escalation of response within the immune system.

On the other hand, undernutrition yields a weaker immune system. Whether it may be a result of food deficits or scarcities in some developing countries, or malnutrition arising due to inflation or intervals of hospitalization in other, the impairment of the immune system would depend upon the severity of the nutrient deficiency, presence of any disorder and age of the deficient.

It is also considered to know that adverse effects on the immune system can occur with the deficiency of just a single nutrient. Such is the case of Vitamin E, which not only acts as an antioxidant, interacts with enzymes, but also helps in transporting proteins. It is also to be contemplated, that excess intake of some micronutrients can also attribute to impaired immune systems. However, researches are still under observation to discern how inevitable nutritional intrusions can enhance immune functions before even the onset of symptoms of a specific infection or disease.

Here I have collected a list of food rich in immune-boosting nutrients. Next time you visit your grocery, don't forget to include them on the list.

1.   Citrus fruit and Vitamin C sources

Even my eight-year-old knows that all citrus fruits contain Vitamin C. It is beneficial in the flu and cold. It helps to reinforce the immune system by aggregating the number of white blood cells, which are the primary agents to fight off any infection. You can easily squeeze them in water or even foods. These citrus fruits include:-

- grapefruit

- oranges

- tangerines

- clementine

- lemons

- limes

For continue balance in nutrition, it is essential to incorporate these foods into your diet because Vitamin C is not produced in our bodies and should be outsourced.

Vitamin C is prominent for healing wounds, repair, and maintenance of healthy bones, skin, teeth, and bone cartilage. It works as an antioxidant and fights with free radicals in our bodies that help in preventing various diseases and facilitate healthy aging. There are no researches that may confirm that Vitamin C would prevent you from cold or flu, but it may delay the symptoms for one or two days for some people.

Besides citrus, many other fruits and vegetables are a source of this fundamental Vitamin. These sources include strawberries, tomatoes, potatoes, green and red peppers, kiwi fruit, papaya, and Brussels sprouts. It is also important to mention that while consuming Vitamin C rich foods, it is vital to eat them fresh, and as soon as you bring them home to reap most of the nutrients out of them.

2.   Broccoli and Leafy Vegetables

Broccoli is a superpower food rich in vitamins and minerals. It is loaded with vitamins A, C, and E, along with lots of fiber and antioxidants. Broccoli is considered one of the healthiest vegetables you can incorporate in your diet.

Studies show that broccoli contains a chemical called sulforaphane, which helps in triggering antioxidants and specific enzymes in immune cells. These cells fight off the destructive effects of free radicals that can damage cells and open doors to various diseases.

Some healthy body functions like the metabolic conversion of food into energy or polluted air results in free radicals inside our bodies. These are highly charged molecules and can inflict tissue damage leading to diseases like clogged arteries. This oxidative damage of the body is considered as the fundamental cause of pre-aging and aging effects.

Retaining a poor balance between these free radicals and antioxidants troops in the body can stipulate the impacts of various illnesses allied with aging that includes diabetes, cardiovascular disease, arthritis as well as deterioration in the effectiveness of the immune system to fight against infectious microorganisms.

Broccoli acts as a blessing to our immune system and anti-aging effects by providing sufficient antioxidants to our bodies. Along with broccoli, spinach and other green vegetables are not only rich in Vitamin C and antioxidants but also contain carotene, which increases the proficiency of our immune system for fighting infections. It is also suggested that to extract maximum nutrients from it. You should look into the cooking procedures and cook it as little as possible or even better eat raw. Studies show that the best way to retain nutrients in vegetables is to steam before consuming them

3.   Nuts

Almost all nuts, including almonds, walnuts, cashews, pistachios, are essential components for working in harmony for the immunity system. They contain Zinc, Iron, copper, selenium, and folate. Chestnuts also contain Vitamin C.

Vitamin E in almonds are high for cold and flu and even tend to outperform Vitamin C. They are a good source of antioxidants, which are the essential components of a healthy immune system.

Walnuts are packed with essential vitamins and minerals that include copper and Vitamin B6. Both these components help in bone health, nerve system, and hence strengthening immunity functions.

Brazil nuts are a nutritious and powerful source for a well-performing immune system. They include selenium, Iron, and Zinc. However, they are distinguished from other nuts as having a high content of selenium. Where it prevents nerve cell damage, it also helps in strengthening the immune system.

A healthy immune system needs an optimum Vitamin B6 consumption. Pistachios are rich in Vitamin B6 and benefit in healthy blood flow, hence oxygen throughout the cells, maintaining healthy lymphoid glands, that is, the spleen, thymus, and the lymph nodes. These are crucial for white blood cell productions that ensure body defense against infections.

The addition of Zinc to your diet can help you fight off your next cold. It is a fundamental component of a robust immune system. Cashew nuts are rich in copper, as well as in Zinc. Scientists reveal that zinc assists in cells of the body to fight infections and maintain immune response balance.

4.   **Garlic**

Garlic is a must in almost every cuisine all around the world. It is a must-have for a healthy lifestyle, and a hint of it gives that tanginess to your taste.

Garlic is rich in antioxidants and has historical significance for fighting infections. It has it's medicinal properties and is also proved beneficial for heart and arteries, flu and colds, and the immune system. Its immune-boosting properties are believed to come from its dense concentration of a compound called Alicen, which is rich in sulfur.

Allicin is produced when you chop, cut, crush or chew garlic and serves with the fighting of virus and bacteria in the blood, mainly associated with flu and colds.

The cooking methods are also in consideration of the medicinal effects of garlic. Crushed and sliced garlic are high in Alicen content. Stand for 10 minutes before cooking your crushed garlic. It prevents the loss of its medicinal behavior. To obtain maximum benefits, use a little more in quantity, more than a clove per meal.

5.   Ginger

Ginger is another world-famous antioxidant, and its consumption is well known for the treatment of stomach ailments and nausea. Antioxidants are elements in our bodies that protect us from withstanding free radicals. They play an integral role in cancer, heart diseases, and other infections.

Ginger also helps decrease inflammation, which helps cure sore throat and inflammatory disorders. It also works as an immunity booster antibiotic that helps reduce pain and infections. It is rich in anti-inflammatory components, which are called gingerol. It is responsible for replacing blood vessels, which, as a result, proves beneficial for chronic asthmatic patients or patients with bronchial infections.

It's also rich in paradol, sesquiterpenes, shogaols, and zingerone. All of which are laden with anti-inflammatory and antioxidant properties. Ginger tea has been used in ancient times in many parts of the world as an immunity strengthening antioxidant drink. Is has a slight pungent herbal smell and works in combatting inflammation externally as well as internally.

Researchers advise that increasing your intake of antioxidant-rich foods and drinks that help fight inflammation keeps your immune system healthy. Ginger shots have become recently popular that are drinks containing ginger extracts with added vitamins, lemons, and herbs. These act as substantial antibiotics and antiviral properties. Ginger detox drinks are also famous for weight loss due to its property of increasing the thermic effect of food, or the calories consumed, which in return helps in strengthening immunity.

6.   **Shellfish**

You may not have thought of Shellfish to be prominent for helping you in strengthening the immune system. But to your surprise, these are rich in zinc mineral.

Zinc is mostly ignored in our significant list of vitamins and minerals, although it is so essential for our immune cells to function correctly. It is to be marked that Zinc is not produced and stored by our bodies, and we have to outsource it from food or supplements.

Shellfish that are rich in Zinc include:

- Crabs

- Lobsters

- Oysters

- Mussels

Zinc is considered as the second, the first on being iron, the most abundant trace mineral in our bodies. It is present and performs excellently in every cell of our bodies. Where Zinc helps to keep our immune system healthy, it is necessary for more than 300 enzymes that contribute to digestion, metabolism, nerve function, and many other body processes that include:

- Reaction of enzymes

- Syntheses of proteins

- Immune function

- Gene expression

- Healing of wounds

- Growth and development

- DNA synthesis

Deficiency of Zinc can lead to weak immune responses, hence promoting the body's tendency to catch viruses and infections. Other than Shellfish, additional food sources like dairy, meat, legumes, seeds, eggs, and poultry are also good sources of Zinc. It is crucial to keep your Zinc levels accurate for healthy performing body systems and immunity.

7.   Yogurt

The probiotic functional properties of yogurt are well known globally. Greek yogurt is richer in Vitamin D and protein that may help in finding infections. Not only consuming yogurt, but it was also used as a medicinal ointment on wounds and infections in ancient times.

Researchers suggest that possessing a healthy level of Vitamin D helps in strengthening your immune system by adequate immune cells functioning, T- cells, and pathogens that help you from fighting off various infections, even contagious ones. It is also proved vital for general respiratory illnesses and can also be helpful in pandemics that affect the lungs.

However, Vitamin D may not be the solution to any pandemic, or it's symptoms, it is necessary to adopt the precautionary measures of social distancing along with working on immune system defense. This Vitamin proves crucial in improving immune responses. Where is works as an anti-inflammatory, it also regulated resistant system properties of fighting infections.

Yogurt and other dairy products such as eggs yolks and cheese are rich in Vitamin D. You can also obtain it from sunlight. Salmon fish is also a great source of this essential Vitamin.

8.   Sunflower seeds

Sunflower seeds are mini nutrient bombs that are loaded up with vitamins and minerals. These include phosphorus, magnesium, folate, selenium, and copper, Zinc, Vitamin B-6, and Vitamin E. All these elements play a crucial role in enhancing the immune system functioning, some of which are discussed previously.

Selenium is a vital component found in sunflower seeds that are proved to combat viral diseases, including contagious ones. It helps our immune system from cell damage and fights your body against cancerous cells. Just a single ounce of these seeds provides half of the daily selenium an average human needs in a day.

Vitamin E has powerful anti-inflammatory properties and reduces the risk of associated heart problems. It is essential for the immune system functioning moreover maintains healthy skin, nails, and hair. Some other food sources of Vitamin E are leafy or green vegetables and also avocados.

These mini bombs are also rich in magnesium that is pertained to hundreds of distinct body functions. This mineral is believed to lower blood pressure, reduce the risk of cardiovascular disease, and controls blood sugar levels. According to a registered American dietician Brain ST. Pierre "It's also a vital component of bone and helps to regulate our nerve and muscle function and contraction."

9.   **Poultry**

I always remember my mom bringing a hot bowl of chicken broth whenever I had caught a cold. It still had been a source of relief and comfort. Mom knew that having a bowl of chicken broth would cure my cold, but less did she know that Vitamin B-6 is the most essential performer that would do the job. Poultry is rich in Vitamin B-6. This Vitamin helps in the formation of healthy and fresh red blood cells. Vitamin B-6 is an essential player in many of the chemical reactions that happen in the body. It benefits the immune systems by decreasing the intensity and duration of cold symptoms by preventing white blood cells from migrating around the mucous membrane; hence, reducing congestion and blockage this aids in reducing inflammation and thus curing severe symptoms. Chicken broth or stock contains gelatine, chondroitin, vitamin A and C, phosphorous, magnesium, and antioxidants, which benefits in healing gut and immunity. It is a thousand times more effective than having just hot water as it thins mucus and speeds its movements in the nose, which reduces the amount of virus attack that may contact with the nose lining and decrease the length of cold. Just about 3 ounces of chicken or turkey includes the daily recommended amount of B-6 Vitamin.

Poultry meat contains amino acids that are building blocks to antibodies that fight off infections. Different cuts of chicken and poultry, and also trying out the liver, will give you a great source of Iron, Zinc, vitamin A and more. It creates a defense system secure against various diseases, including cancer and infectious diseases.

THE BOTTOM LINE

Food undoubtedly plays a vital role in the strengthening of our immune system, but it should be made sure that you have everything fresh and healthy. Avoid high-calorie foods, and it is usually suggested to consume 30 to 60 grams of healthy carbs during physical activity, thus maintaining a healthy immune system.

CHAPTER 3

ROLE OF VITAMINS AND MINERALS SUPPLEMENTS FOR A HEALTHY IMMUNE SYSTEM

Studies have proven that people' connected with nature' are said to be stronger and healthier, having increased life span with less susceptibility to infections. They barely fall prey to diseases owing to their better immune system, which is fuelled bt nature in the form of food, providing necessary nutrients to the body, including vitamins.

Vitamins, also called micronutrients, are needed in small quantities, which play a crucial role in providing energy for maintenance of body processes, i.e., strengthening bones, healing wounds, repairing cell damage, and upgrading the immune system. They are termed as 'essential' as the body does not synthesize them; hence they are taken externally. It is also virtuous to know that you cannot build your immune system by eating four oranges all at once. These habits are developed over time by maintaining healthy eating procedures throughout your life.

The term 'connected with nature' symbolically relates to the consumption of raw food, e.g., fruits, vegetables, dairy products, etc. which are the best possible sources other than pills. Being organic in nature and obtained by plants and animals, they are often destroyed or rendered ineffective when cooked or processed.

So, even if you consume the healthiest and balanced diet, but the cooking procedures are not checked or appropriately followed, you can end up in nutrient deficient. The deficiency of vitamins presents a weaker immune system prone to numerous infections and imminent diseases. As we have already discussed dominant vitamins and minerals that play a vital role in maintaining our immune system, let us also disclose the effects of their deficiency in our bodies.

Taking into consideration the intake of vitamins, you should also know that where we are ingesting Vitamins, these are also excreted. Vitamins are mainly divided into two categories, water-soluble vitamins and fat-soluble vitamins depending upon their solubility. Water-soluble vitamins are soluble in water, thus are excreted with urine hence frequently needed. These include Vitamin C and Vitamin B family.

Fat-soluble vitamins are stored as reserves in the liver and tissues. These include Vitamin A, D, E, and K. These vitamins provide decent repairs to various organs and systems. Should be consumed by doctor's recommendations.

1.   Vitamin C

You already know that you can obtain most of your vitamin C from citrus fruits and many of the leafy green vegetables. You may not need to take extra supplements for it if you are following daily dietary sources, or you can consult your doctor for any of its deficiency symptoms in your body. It is a water-soluble vitamin so you can get deficient in it if not outsourced from food.

Vitamin C is involved in many processes of the immune system and boosts the white blood cell production within the cells. It directly enhances the production of lymphocytes and phagocytes, which are the protective agents against microbes and infectious diseases.

As they also act defensive for free radicals, it performs as an antioxidant and shortens the healing time of wounds. It is researched that people showing pneumonia symptoms tend to have lesser Vitamin C levels, and keeping them on Vitamin C supplements have shortened their recovery time.

Scurvy, a gum disease, and less immunity to colds and flu are symptoms of Vitamin C deficiency. Some other symptoms may include dry skin and hair, bleeding gums, nosebleeds, problems in coping with infections and healing wounds, joint pains.

2.   Vitamin E

Vitamin E is an antioxidant and protects cells from free radicals and cell damage, protecting against infections and viruses hence a crucial element during pandemics. It may also aid in lowering various risks of health problems that include heart diseases, cancer, and probably even dementia.

Seeds, nuts, and food sources are discussed above for this Vitamin. Where deficiency of Vitamin E causes weak immunity, it also causes muscle and nerve damage that show loss of movement in the body along with the loss of feeling in arms and legs.

Vitamin E is fat-soluble. It is quite rare to be deficient in this Vitamin unless you show some primary health conditions like difficulty in coordination or walking, visual imbalance, weakness or muscle pain, weak immune system, and catching infections for often.

The recommended dietary allowance (RDA) of Vitamin E for over the age of 14 is 15milligrams. Women who breastfeed may need a little more that is 19mg. As it is not on a more excellent range, doses less than 1000mg are safe for most adults.

Being a fat-soluble vitamin, it is not excreted through urine. It means if over consumed, it can accumulate to toxic levels over time. Some overdose symptoms include nausea, fatigue, blurred or low vision, headaches, migraines, rashes, or even gonadal dysfunction.

3.   Vitamin B-6

Vitamin B-6 is known as pyridoxine and is one of the vitamins in the B complex group. It is crucial for more than a hundred and fifty enzyme reactions in the body. It is associated with the chief functions of your immune and nervous systems and also helps with your body procedure of protein, carbs, and fat that you consume.

If following a healthy diet plan, most people can obtain enough of B6 from their diet alone. But if you have low levels of other B complex Vitamins like B12 or folate, then you might more likely be deficient in Vitamin B6 too. This deficiency is observed in people familiar with liver, digestive, kidney, or autoimmune diseases and also smokers, alcoholics, overweight people, and pregnant women.

Vitamin B6 has antioxidant and anti-inflammatory properties, thus help in strengthening immunity and also preventing chronic conditions like cancer and heart diseases.

Preventing inflammation, infections, and various types of cancer are the key to having a well-functioning immune system. Deficiency of B6 can disturb the working of the immune system resulting in lower anti-bodies production required to fight infections. It also reduces white blood cell production along with T-cells that regulate immune function, helping it to respond correctly. Increased destruction of this Vitamin is found in people with the disorder in their autoimmune system, which increases their demand for Vitamin B6.

Sources of Vitamin B6 are mainly meat like turkey, chicken, pork, steak, and fish. Some fruits like avocadoes and bananas, sunflower seeds, prunes, and boiled lentils are sources other than meat. Markedly, sources of B6 from animal and fortified foods along with supplements are absorbed better than plant food forms. So, if you are a vegetarian, you may need to make up the deficiency of B6 in your body.

Introducing a variety of meat, fruits, and vegetables in your diet can quickly meet up your Vitamin B6 needs. Still, some symptoms of its deficiency may include skin rashes, mood changes, glossy tongue, impaired immune system, tiredness, elevated homocysteine levels, and seizures.

If you are worried that you may not be consuming enough of Vitamin B6 food sources, or you are showing some deficiency symptoms, it is best to talk to your doctor for the best action to be taken. One can quickly get B6 deficiency as long as you have wholesome eating habits. In some severe cases of symptoms, supplements for B-complex or B6 may be advised.

4.   Vitamin A

Go rainbow with Vitamin A. These are mostly colorful fruits and vegetables called carotenoids. Some bright examples are carrots, sweet potatoes, cantaloupe, pumpkin, and squash. These carotenoids are turned into Vitamin A by our bodies that act as antioxidants and help strengthen our immune system fighting infections. Vitamin A, when obtained from animal sources, is called retinol. Animal sources include beef liver, lamb liver, cod liver oil, salmon, goat cheese, hard-boiled eggs, and butter.

Vitamin A is also fat-soluble Vitamin hence easily dissolved in fats and oils. It can be stored in the body if consumed too much and has toxic effects. Vitamin A is crucial for all life processes and plays a vital role in fighting off infections. It prevents dryness of skin and hence strengthening the immune system. Vitamin A is crucial for the treatment of infectious diseases like tuberculosis, measles, AIDS, and other infectious diseases in children.

Deficiency of Vitamin A shows some severe symptoms like dry skin and dry eyes, night blindness, delayed growth, slow wound healing, throat and chest infections, and many prone to pandemics. If you are diagnosed with Vitamin A deficiency, your doctor will recommend supplements and will ask you to watch your diet. Most doctors will suggest retinol instead of beta-carotene.

5.   VITAMIN D

As mentioned, it is best to get your Vitamins from food; Vitamin D is the exception to this rule. You can enhance your intake of food, but many people find it difficult, absorbing Vitamin D from food sources. Some of the food sources are fatty fish like salmon, tuna, sardines and mackerel, and some fortified foods like cereals, milk, and orange juice.

Vitamin D is also obtained from sunlight at various times of the day, and it is also called the "sunshine Vitamin." It is a fat-soluble vitamin and consists of Vitamin D family of D-1, D-2, and D-3. Vitamin D has many crucial functions, the most important of which are the phosphorus and calcium absorption to facilitate the immune system's normal functioning. Along with resistance against certain diseases, it is also vital for normal body functioning and growth and development of healthy bones and teeth.

Vitamin D is essential to keep our immune system stay in balance. It tends to work as a backup for keeping us healthy, especially during the flu and cold season. On the exterior of all white blood cells are located, enzymes that are used for activation along with Vitamin D receptors. Vitamin D is vital to keep the immune system operate with proper balance. Due to increased stimulation, the autoimmune system can get started and inactivity of the immune system that can result in regular infections and illness.

Although lower levels of Vitamin D may not be the underlying cause of autoimmune disease, it can make the condition to worsen. According to the National Institute of Health, lesser levels of Vitamin D are accompanying severe conditions of colds and influenza. Since their announcement, many studies have been determined to recognize this association and proved that Vitamin D is crucial for fighting disease.

A simple blood test is done to diagnose a deficiency of Vitamin D in your body. If it is traced, then your doctor would do your X-rays to check your bone strength. Vitamin D supplements are advised with low levels of this Vitamin, and in some severe cases, high doses of liquids or tablets are given.

According to International Units (IUs) per day, the recommended doses of Vitamin D are 600IU for children under 18, adults till 70, and pregnant women. Older people above 70 should have 800IU per day.

6.   IRON

Iron is one of the fundamental elements for the healthy development of the immune system. It is necessary for the production and growth of immune cells, mainly the production of lymphocytes, which are associated with the creation of exceptional response to infections. It is also used to make red blood cells that transport oxygen to all the other parts of the body, making it imperative for all body systems to work in order.

Iron is essential for the production of parasites, bacteria, and neoplastic cells, saying so an excess of this element could potentially enable the growth of cells causing infections and, thus, tumors. Our immune system has a mechanism that reduces the availability of iron that promotes the growth of bacteria. It is called a bacteriostatic mechanism. Iron is used as a transitional metal in the production of theses bacteriostatic cells by our immune system. It is, therefore, essential to have a check that high levels of iron can, on the other hand, suppress that immune.

However, if Iron deficiency is ignored, it can make you more vulnerable to illness and infections. Lack of Iron acts negatively at the body's natural defense system. Iron deficiency is called anemia and causes various heart diseases.

Its symptoms show shortness of breath, lack of energy, or pale complexion.

Some good food sources of iron include red meat, seafood, animal liver, chicken, and turkey. For vegetarians, they can get their metal from beans, broccoli, spinach, and kale.

7.   ZINC

Zinc, a trace mineral, plays a crucial role in the body, and it can be obtained through various food sources and supplements. It cannot be deposited in the body, so it is recommended to induce its regular intake. Zinc is needed for different chemical reactions in our body that includes almost 300 enzyme chemical reactions. It is also required for various metabolism and growth reactions, protein synthesis, and skin health, healing of wounds, DNA synthesis, fertility, digestion, and hormonal balance, sense of smell and taste, and also immunity.

Deficiency of Zinc in the body causes a weaker immune system altogether. It malfunctions the inborn and adaptive immune system leaving our body incapable of protecting itself from harmful viruses and bacteria. Its deficiency also causes inflammation in the body and shows a role in dermatitis, inflammatory bowel diseases, or arthritis. It is likewise proved by the researchers that Zinc supplements help in reducing the sternness and period of cold and flu indications when administered at the first symptoms in 24 hours.

Food sources of Zinc are oysters, pumpkins seeds, red meat, ginger root, beans and legumes, fish and seafood, whole wheat, dairy products, eggs, and chocolate. Its daily recommended dose for men is 9.5mg/day, women 7mg/day, 12mg/day for pregnant women, and 13mg/day for breastfeeding women.

This element is vital for the immune system to fight off infections. You may need to add a zinc supplement in your regime if you are a vegetarian or don't like to eat meat. People with various illnesses like diabetes, digestive problems, sickle cell anemia, and liver disorders may not be able to absorb Zinc from food.

THE BOTTOM LINE

While mentioning all these benefits of micronutrients, it is also essential to discuss that overdosing on these or any of the Vitamins or Minerals may prove counterproductive or even play a reverse role for the immune system to function correctly. For instance, Iron supplementation can enhance fatality for those residing in malaria-endemic zones. There is, however, extensive research on nutrition as the primary cause of weak immunity and supplements can benefit effectively in treating immune deficiencies due to inadequate intake. Furthermore, the intervention of these micronutrients can enhance immune functions, especially in subclinical symptoms, preventing the commencement of infectious or chronic inflammatory diseases.

CHAPTER 4

WATER, WATER, WATER!

Truly water is a magical element for all body functions to keep going and crucial for immune system functioning too. It benefits the natural health of a body by its miraculous properties. Water is essential in transferring substances throughout the body. It supports the immune system directly as well as indirectly to help keep its army healthy and defensive and available for the enemies (microbes) day in and day out.

Immune function is an essential biological process that can be suppressed due to the deficiency of various resources while they are used up by other physical tasks in the body. Water is particularly a helpful resource profoundly used by all bodily functions that can result in a lack of availability for other primary services. Regardless, its osmotic state on immune functions is much of a concern for the accomplishment of various functions of combating germs and infections.

Gulping on some enough water to keep you hydrated in important at a daily routine, especially during the flu and cold season. To keep yourself away from infections, it is a great idea to prevent yourself from dehydration. Staying hydrated prevents you from detoxifying your body and eliminate germs and bacteria that may accumulate and therefore cause infections. Recommended eight ounces per day should be taken, and even more, if you are exercising or during hot weather.

Water plays a huge role in almost all of the chief cellular functions of an organism, mainly, which includes mobile volume and its composition, heat shock protein production, plasma hormone concentration, development of cells, and membrane permeability. Due to a change in osmotic state, it may affect abundant phases of various functions in the body, also susceptible to influence the accurate functioning of the immune system.

Our human body is made up of 75% of water, and you may know that we can survive for just a week without water. While in a state of dehydration, it becomes difficult for our system to remove toxins and waste from our body, and it becomes more vulnerable to infections and diseases.

Furthermore, it lowers energy levels, which results in weak metabolism and hence a weakened immune system.

A study was designed on astronauts and athletes that proved a drop in their immune system due to different stress that they experienced during extended flights. Dehydration is one of the everyday stressors for both athletes and astronauts. It exposed the role of hydration and the effects it placed on the immune system. This study proved that the concentration of electrolytes called Plasma osmolality tends to be the guiding force for the immune system rather than plasma volume. It demonstrates that it is essential to preserve proper osmolality for athletes and astronauts with appropriate hydration.

Therefore to maintain the right amounts of salts and electrolytes in the body for better immune functioning, it is crucial to have an adequate resource of water. Dehydration may also cause cellular as well as emotional stress than also affects the operation of the immune system and hence a higher tendency to catch infectious diseases.

You can add up water in the form of soups, broths, green tea, herbal drinks, or fruit juices. You can similarly add lemon or honey to your pool and make it an energy booster that may keep you active and robust, building up immunity against antibodies and infectious diseases.

CHAPTER 5

HERBS AND IMMUNITY

It is often seen during a pandemic or viral season, even when all your friends and fellows may get affected, some may still stand tall and healthy. Ever thought about how some people often get sick while others stay in good condition, even in the flu and cold season? It all depends on the person's immune system and how much he takes care of it. As you already know that our body consists of our defense system against infectious illnesses. Although it is a naturally healthy body process, you can work on it to function efficiently against aliens that would invade your body and make you sick.

Since ancient times many herbs and plants had medicinal properties and are proved effective in fighting against viruses and bacteria or even prevent them from attacking our bodies. These herbs, being natural, are safe to use and do not have any side effects like other allopathic. Herbs like Echinacea, Andrographis, Elderberry, AHCC are to name some. Let us now discuss some of the most popular and proven herbs that work best to make your defense system healthier and even help you cure after you would have been got attacked. At the end of this chapter, we have also mentioned a proven herbal recipe for a more robust immune system used in China during the recent pandemic.

1.   ROSEMARY

Rosemary is used in cooking as well but also has healing properties due to its plant compound that includes oleanolic acid. Antiviral applications of oleanolic acid are proved against HIV, herpes virus, influenza, and hepatitis. Moreover, rosemary extracts are beneficial in liver diseases, like herpes viruses and hepatitis A.

How to use it?

- Add a few rosemary leaves, dried or fresh, in boiling water, stew for some time, and enjoy this antiviral drink sip by sip. You can add some honey.

- Rosemary springs can be added to meats and dishes for flavor and health.

- Few drops of rosemary extract can be used in your steamer for a deep inhalation through your nose.

- It can be used in your humidifier, or you can also add a few drops in your room spray.

- You can also use its oil directly, mixing a few drops with olive or coconut oil, as it can be a bit strong all by itself.

- You can also mix a few drops of the extract with your body lotion or moisturizer.

- Add some drops in your bathtub and enjoy antiviral cleansing.

2. Echinacea

Echinacea is quite a popular ingredient in the herbal world of medicine because of its remarkable properties in promoting health and preventing illness. Almost all of its parts, flowers, leaves, and roots are useful for natural medicinal remedies.

One of its variety, Echinacea purpura that grows the native Americans widely used a cone-shaped flower for various purposes and viral infections. Multiple studies prove that these flowers are significantly useful in fighting off viral infections that include herpes and influenza

Echinacea purpura itself has immune-boosting effects hence useful for infectious treatments. It is particularly effective in upper respiratory tract infections and for treating wounds topically.

Products like juice, teas, and tablets are available in the market to use in different ways. Extracts are also available, and it is used by adding just a few drops in some quantity of water for the healing of specific conditions according to the instructions.

## 3.	PEPPERMINT

Peppermint and its extracts are famous in naturally treating viral infections and inflammation. An active compound like methanol and rosmarinic acid in its leaves and essential oils act as antiviral against diseases and are added to teas and tinctures for treatment of wounds or inflammation.

A researched test-tube study shows that peppermint leaf extract act as a potent antiviral against RSV (respiratory syncytial virus) and for various anti-inflammatory infections. Due to its anti-inflammatory properties, peppermint oil aids in clearing air passages and reduces snoring and helps you have a calm sleep, which directly affects your immunity. It is also proved useful in common colds and being anti-fungal, anti-bacterial for various illnesses, and building immunity.

Peppermint essential oils are quite healthy, so few drops are used with other carrier oils for massaging or used in sprays and bathtubs. Peppermint leaves are used as a food flavoring in Indian and South Asian cuisines and for various stomach related problems used as tea leaves or in dried form.

4. ASTRAGALUS

This flowering herb is popular in traditional Chinses herbal medicine. Its main ingredient, Astragalus polysaccharide APS has potent anti-inflammatory, antiviral, and immune-enhancing qualities. It does not only help to prevent various illnesses but is also used for the treatment of multiple diseases like the common cold, fibromyalgia, upper respiratory infections, and diabetes.

Astragalus is abundantly used in China for viral infections pandemics, but it has not proven to cure it. However, animal studies and test-tube show that it is fruitful in combating herpes viruses, avian influenza H9 virus, and hepatitis C. It also demonstrates that APS protects human astrocyte cells, which are the primary cells of the central nervous system.

Astragalus is rich in antioxidant effects, prevents the production of free radicals, and works in harmony with your immune system. It is also castoff as a nutritional supplement for various health conditions and combats weaknesses due to infections. Its benefits are extracted by its leaves tea or root tea available in the market. Also available in the form of oil and tablets.

5.   GINSENG

Ginseng is a root of a plant of the family Panax, which is mostly found in American and Korean family. Is has been used as Chinese herbal medicine in ancient times, and has been proven potent for treating viral infections. It is an antioxidant and anti-inflammatory, helps regulate sugar levels in the body, and works wonders for some cancers like stomach cancers.

This miraculous root works wonders with the immune system and lower reappearance of symptoms due to its role in T-cell proliferation. It is recognized worldwide to strengthen the immune system, fight fatigue, boost brain functions, and improve symptoms of erectile dysfunction.

Studies suggest that people who use ginseng regularly have a higher chance of living disease-free lives and have a higher endurance rate when compared to people not taking it. Moreover, people have recovered from stomach cancer surgery by using 5,400mg daily for two years.

Some studies show the effect of red ginseng extract on the immune system that helps enhance the impact of vaccinations and diseases such as influenza and common colds. It is also effective against viral attacks like RSV and hepatitis A. Ginesenoisides compound in ginseng is effective against hepatitis B, norovirus, and several other bacterial infections as well.

It is available in various forms in the market as immune booster herbal tea extract, tables, and supplements, oil, oral drops, balms or lotions.

6.   ELDERBERRY

Elderberry, from Sambucus tree, consists of many varieties that have bunches of white flowers on them with black or blue-black berries. The commonly used type for herbal medicinal use is Sambucus nigra, which is also known as blackberry or European elderberry.

Elderberry has been used in history for medicinal and culinary purposes. Recommended by doctors worldwide, it works as an antioxidant, antiviral, and anti-inflammatory herb. Anciently, its flowers and leaves have been used for relieving pain, inflammation, swelling, stimulant to urine production, and sweat induction. Its bark was used as a laxative and induced nausea and vomiting.

Traditionally, dried berries or their juice is used to treat infections, influenza, sciatica, headaches, heart, and dental pain, and also used as laxative and diuretic. Packed with vitamins and antioxidants also support the enhancement of your immune system. The berries may also be cooked to make jams, pies, juices, and elderberry wine. They can be used fresh and consumed raw, or the flowers are often stewed with sugar and water for infused tea with medicinal properties.

Elderberry has vast uses and forms, and it is also found in a variety of syrups, tablets, gummies, pills, and teas. Entirely safe to use, it is also used as food coloring, body lotions, balms, and cosmetics. It can be induced as a part of a healthy diet plan, along with the use of other vitamins and supplements.

THE BOTTOM LINE

Herbs have been used since ancient times as natural remedies for several diseases and immunity strengthening as they have very few to no side effects. It is also advisable to encourage the use of shared kitchen herbs like oregano, basil, sage, thyme, and even some rare herbs like Sambuca's and astragalus have potent impacts on microbes than invade human bodies hence causing it to fight against infection.

They can easily be used by adding aroma and zest to your recipes or just sipping as herbal antioxidant teas. However, although having a variety of benefits and researches, it cannot be confirmed if such small doses of beneficial herbs could have similar effects. To enjoy complete advantage of these natural immunity boosters as supplements, extracts, herbal products, oils, or syrups. It would be safe to consult your health provider for safe and beneficial use of dosage.

CHAPTER 6

EXERCISE AND ITS EFFECTS ON IMMUNITY

Exercise has many benefits other than making us fit and increasing our strength. Exercising is good, mentally, and physically. Intellectually speaking, it makes us stress-free and releases hormones like dopamine and endorphins that make us feel happy, light-headed, relaxed, and joyous. Physical changes are pretty noticeable; your muscle builds up, and you cut down some fat. The unique phenomenon that occurs in our body during exercise is with our immune system. To understand how it affects our immune system, let's figure out how our body acts during exercise.

Exercise pushes your body to your physical threshold, and a consistent pace help to increase that the limit. Workout pushes our body to the extreme, which can result in many complications if not done correctly. But, there are some complications that everyone faces because of exercising and that are sore muscles. Muscles become sore because of the accumulation of lactic acid that is released during anaerobic respiration. Lactic acids make our muscles stiffs, but this is not the whole story. Our muscles get micro-tears that are not visible to us, but our robust immune system quickly rushes to the site of damage and repairs it.

It is the role of the immune system in exercise, but does the immune system is boosted with use. The simple answer is unsettling. In response to activity, there is an immune response, which is a healthy immune response. Researchers at the University of Bath of exercise physiology and immunobiology, U.K., reports that it is probably more accurate to say exercise stimulates or kicks off some normal immune processes instead of boosting. Here's what's going on: when you engage in any kind of physical activity that will increase your heart rate for a sustained amount of time. From bike riding to proper body training, your body interoperates it as physiological stress, which lets your body to move certain types of white blood cells, which includes neutrophils and lymphocytes (particularly T-cells and natural killer cells) from different parts of your lymphatic system to flood your bloodstream. Because of their presence, they kill any potential threat from their body cleansing from the cure. This vast quantity also helps to get rid of cancer-causing cells as well. That is why it is said that exercise prevents cancer.

Immune cells begin to decrease and even go down into below-average levels in your bloodstream shortly after your workout. Scientists initially claimed that this was proof of immunosuppression (dampening of the body's ability to combat infection and disease), but it's not true. Better laboratory methods revealed that such cells were only transported to other body locations where the mechanism of immune response is continued. They are passed to other tissues in the body, such as the lungs or even the skin, gut, or mucus, where there is a higher chance of infection. Each sudden boost in immunity lasts for about three hours but can be experienced after a round of any type of exercise. If you exercise daily, you will experience this phenomenon daily. It keeps your immune system active and regulating.

Evidence has shown that people who frequently exercise results get sick less often. According to a 2010 article in the British Journal of Sports Medicine, reported that people who exercised for at least 20 minutes a day, five or more days per week, reported 43% fewer days with respiratory and lung infection symptoms than those who were inactive and dozing on the couch. And when they did get sick, their indications were not severe or out of control. It doesn't mean that you cannot get infected at all if you exercise; it helps your immune system by no means it makes you invincible or immortal.

The most hotly debated topic in the relation of the immune system and exercise is that, Can Too Much Exercise Decrease Your Immunity? Many athletes fell ill after 90 minutes of vigorous practicing. They usually experience some respiratory problems. Their reports do mention that exercising can be a cause of this, but they never mention the white blood cells count in there study, causing confusion and delusion in the society. The illness comes down to the environment they are practicing in if you run a marathon and fallen ill. It's not because you have overdone yourself; it's probably because of the environment you were in. What were you inhaling during the run, these types of factors are deducted from the reports. These reports are mainly based on observation rather than actual research. Because there is misperception regarding this topic, the answer to this question cannot be answered. But, we can say that exercising for an hour is perfect. If you really want to push yourself, then workout in an optimum environment instead of a dusty garage or a sandy road.

Exercising is vital for your immune system. If you don't work out at all, your immune system becomes lazy with you meaning they lost their effectiveness, making you prone to illnesses and inflammations. It will be useful, but you will not have an extra shield of protection around your body. You don't need a proper gym membership and a 60-minute schedule to become invulnerable to small infections, a 15 to 30-minute jog or anything that accelerates your heartbeat can help you get better immunity.

CHAPTER 7

HAZARDOUS EFFECTS OF SMOKING ON IMMUNE SYSTEM

Smoking is the primary cause of preventable deaths all around the world. Tobacco use raises one likelihood of contracting several adverse health problems, some of which may be deadly, as well as leading to the near exposure to other people & ill health, such as relatives and friends. According to many studies, it has been shown that a smoker is more likely to visit a hospital than an average person, even if he is suffering from the common flu, he can require acute attention in the hospital.

Do you know the actual cause of cancer because of Smoking? Only a few of the ingredients involved in a cigarette causes cancer. There are more compounds engaged in; it weakens the immune response, which allows the cancer cells to go unchecked or undefeated by our body and cause deadly cancers. Smoking not only raises the chance of dying, but the likelihood of having certain chronic disorders such as heart problems, stroke, and can also cause complications in reproductive organs, especially in men. Besides, the lungs can also get impacted due to smoke inhalation, which leads to chronic obstructive pulmonary disease (COPD) and pneumonia.

Smoking can aggravate pre-existing breathing conditions, including asthma, bronchitis, and the common cold. Smoking does relieve our stress, but at what cost. While tobacco and cigarette carcinogens are responsible for raising cancer risk, many other compounds perform as pro-inflammatory and immune suppressants agents, including nicotine, formaldehyde, ammonia, carbon monoxide, benzopyrene, tar, acetone, hydroxyquinone, cadmium, and nitrogen oxide. Nicotine is known to be immunosuppressive, which can lead to decreased phagocytic neutrophilic activity and affect chemotaxis and cell signaling, in addition to inhibiting the release of reactive oxygen species (ROS), thus impairing neutrophils & ability to kill pathogens.

Smoking activates a sequence of lung inflammatory agents in which macrophages lead to tissue degradation and further release of inflammatory agents, which lead to persistent chronic inflammatory syndrome. For instance, when triggered, macrophages release interleukin-1, which results in the activation and proliferation of helper-T cells, which trigger killer-T cells themselves. The macrophages in smokers' lungs have a reduced ability for inflammatory phagocytosis agents and dying cells within the lung.

Tregs play a crucial role in their immunosuppressive capacity in maintaining immunological homeostasis and tolerance. Epidemiologic studies also shown that smoking cigarettes in COPD patients can cause Tregs imbalance. Smoking destroys our immune system and makes us prone to diseases that rational human beings would not be endangered. Cigarette smoking impairs Tregs & immunosuppressive activity by decreasing the number of suppressive Tregs or growing the prevalence of non-suppressive Tregs, contributing to an increased autoimmune portion in COPD pathogenesis. In contrast, individual smokers may report increased Treg numbers, contributing to exacerbated respiratory infections. Further in-depth research is required to identify specifically the net impacts of cigarette smoking on Treg generation and work of smokers with or without a particular medical condition.

Cigarette smoking is expected to destroy the immune system & memory cells, ruining the immunity that you developed over the years. Cigarette smoking appeared to dampen rather than strengthen the reaction of children & T-cells by suppressing their generation, a common side effect of passive Smoking.

Exposure to second-hand smoke reduced effector and memory T cells in the lungs and spleens of mycobacterium tuberculosis-infected mice, demonstrating suppressive effects of cigarette smoke on immune responses to infection. Nicotine is an immunosuppressive agent able to modulate innate and adaptive immune responses by communicating with nAChRs on the immune cell surface. But this caused inflammation throughout the body, which can lead to some lifetime complications. But further studies are still required because over the strengthened immune system can cause Autoimmune Disorders, such as rheumatoid arthritis and formation of blood clots.

Nevertheless, in either case, Smoking does play a harmful rather than beneficial role. Tobacco smoke likely emitted from various parts of the world that vary in specific chemical components. It is not clear that Smoking is often dangerous rather than helpful, particularly though it has double effects on immune responses. Cigarette smoke, for example, typically weakens tolerance to pathogens but, paradoxically, encourages autoimmunity. We suspect that with sustained persistent infection, the decreased immunity results in cross-reactive autoimmunity against both a pathogen and a cross-reactive self-tissue.

In the context of various regional immunopathology and diseases, it is also possible that cigarette smoke has differential effects on immunity. While previous studies have revealed some of the cellular and molecular mechanisms responsible for cigarette smoke-induced immunoregulation, the precise mechanisms underlying smoking-associated immunopathology remain mostly unclear. Still, as you might have guessed, further research is required.

Many data prove the adverse effects of smoking Tabaco and how it ruins your life and the life of the people around you. The research supporting the use of cigarettes and other tobacco substance is minute and have a loophole to create confusion among the researchers. So, we cannot say that if nicotine boosts your immune system, it's okay because, as mentioned above, it can cause some other complications as well.

In general, not just tobacco but inhaling any smoke can cause some serious complications as well. Sometimes these smoke from the car and other vehicles if inhaled directly can bind with your red blood cells, making you oxygen deprived, which makes your plasma thicker and cause your immune system to stop working correctly. If you are a smoker and want your immune system to thrive, you probably should think to stop this addiction.

If you are not a smoker and want to prevent yourself from these hazardous effects, then avoid passive Smoking and wear a mask in a crowded area, especially where there is traffic jam almost every day. Preparing yourself for the future pandemic is nothing to be ashamed of. As told, the epidemic is very unpredictable and can kill hundreds of people, and diminishing some activities to increase your chances of survival from any disease is nothing but complimentary.

CHAPTER 8

AGE AND IMMUNITY

The human body is always changing, and these changes lead to aging. Our body is a machine that has its peak point and starts to get rusty over time. Let's begin with why do we age...... for some, aging is the process of growing up, but for others, it means to grow old. This difference in philosophies makes it harder to grasp a single definition of aging. But what we can say is, aging occurs when intrinsic processes and interaction with the environment cause changes in the structure and function of the body's molecules and cells. These factors drive their decline, and overtime causes failure and in our term death. Aging is still a mystery to scientists, but we do know it's effects on the immune system.

When you are an infant, you are prone to diseases, but when you are detached from your mother's placenta, your body gets plenty of antibodies enough to fight off any infection. Then through mother's feed, you start to get antibodies in your system that help your body to develop properly while protecting your internal organs from harmful microbes. An infant's body is learning and adapting. If a baby is exposed to too many infections, it will get resistance from all of the viruses as long as they are not life-threatening. But your bodies learn and overtime everything gets better. During our toddler ages, vaccines work the best because our immune system is developing, which makes it more qualified and defensive.

Your teenage days are your prime time not only for being calm and adventurous but also for your internal body. We all know that we go through some bizarre changes in that time, but the most important thing that happens is that our white blood cells mature. They become more resilient and start to develop immunity from almost every microbe we encounter. It is the age where most of us receive a booster dose, which helps our immune system to work more appropriately.

During our twenties to forties, our immune system stops developing and become more professional in its work. It is quick and completes the job quickly, and it makes rational decisions giving proper outputs. During this age, our immune system is in prime-age because it has learned a lot from its past experiences, and from that, it gets rid of new infections as well. During this time, many people get cured of their allergies as well. But in ages older than forty, things take a huge turn.

All the changes in the human history, in all pandemics and epidemics, scientist notice that people older than 50 – 65 has the higher chance of fatality, this is because during this period of life your immune system starts to degrade. As we grow old, our immune system becomes less effective. Even though the ability of the body to produce white blood cells and antibodies remains the same, the cell's ability to communicate with each other deteriorate. It makes them moves randomly when they get a signal to attack, and as a result, they become less responsive. With time for an unknown reason, your immune system gets blind. They cannot distinguish themselves from microbes and starting attacking themselves. Not only that, but it starts to attack the body as well, which causes autoimmune disorders. It is another reason why diseases like rheumatoid arthritis are more common in old peoples than younger generations.

This miscommunication makes the macrophages that ingest microbes and other foreign cells that help to destroy cancerous cells etc. to slow down. It means that before they work like PacMan and eat bacteria, but as we grow old, it becomes lazy and doesn't work correctly. Similarly, your T-Cells and memory cells that work as an archive system of the body. T-cells have the information about the microbe, and memory cells have the information to kill them. In 65-year-old men, it was seen that there was less production of these cells, which indicates that their immunity was degrading. They were not as immune from an influenza virus (flu virus), then they were in their prime. Which also proves the higher death ratio of older adults from pneumonia.

Now because of less production of T-cells, fewer white blood cells are capable of responding to new antigen, which makes you prone to further infections that your body hasn't encountered yet or any novel virus. Some people think that it is a good thing because you will get fewer allergy attacks. People believe this because allergens are processed as antigens as well. But, beforehand, you take a bite of that Shellfish. It is better to be tested because, in some cases, food allergies become worse in old age. So, always meet a physician if there is your life on the line. Older individuals do not contain as many proteins as younger persons in reaction to bacterial infections provide lower levels of supplementary protein.

Although there is still about the same number of antigens generated, the antibodies are less able to bind to the antigen. This change can partly account for the more common causes of pneumonia, influenza, infectious endocarditis, and tetanus among older people that lead to death. Such improvements will also illustrate in part why vaccinations are less successful in older people and why booster shots (available for certain vaccines) are essential for older adults.

These modifications in the immune system may make older people become more vulnerable to other diseases and cancers. But there is nothing to be scared of, a balanced diet and a healthy body can fight off illnesses that we used to think we can't. With this pandemic on hand, we have seen people age 90 and 80 being cured miraculously because of their proper living standards. Just have a decent lifestyle, eat and drink at the same time and have adequate rest and sleep. Just relax and move around a little to make yourself and healthy and undefeatable.

CHAPTER 9

YOGA AND THE IMMUNE SYSTEM

It is well recognized that people who most often suffer from symptoms of cold and flu, sniffing and sneezing are most of the time people with busy working schedule and overloaded work hours. In other words, they are stressed out, or they have been pushing themselves too hard. According to a study at Bastyr University, naturopathic therapeutics disclose that our body already consists of many silent viruses and bacteria that remain unharmed until something in our body disturbs the equilibrium. Once they get triggered by a raider, they get into action and start to attack. It is crucial to relieve your body from stress in which yoga plays an essential role in facilitating a more robust immune system.

Yoga helps to stay quiet and focused and helps to create empathy towards others and your inner self. You may ask yourself during these panic generating times, that how can one stay calm and make wise decisions. The best way for it is to use the tools available at your ease, keeping your head fresh and practicing mindfulness that lessens emotional reactivity and makes better choices. Time to turn to our ancestors' practices for a better living that has been illustrated to help us maintain a healthy lifestyle.

Consequently, people who regularly practice yoga therapy attests that asana practice can be a day to day means of naturally supporting and strengthening the immune system. Where yoga would help lower stress hormones that negotiate with the immune system, it also habituates the respiratory tract and the lungs while expelling toxins from the body due to the stimulation of the lymphatic system. It also pumps optimal blood to different organs, thereby ensuring preeminent functioning of them. Yoga does not work like routine exercise that work only on specific body parts. It works on the whole body, stretching and relaxing it on the whole and the mind as well.

A yoga practitioner, Mitchell teacher of Paramukta Yoga, which is the "Yoga of Supreme Freedom," demonstrates a plethora of poses that help an executor cure from the winter cold. Another posture, Kurmasana, the tortoise pose, supports the thymus. Adho Mukha Svanasana, which is the Downward-Facing Dog, is beneficial for blood flow through the sinuses. Mitchell also ensures that most of the inverted postures or bending frontward focus the immune system on the sinuses, which in turn helps to relax sinuses. These unique poses also help the preventing of draining lungs along with the associated problems of secondary infections caused due to it.

Ustrasana (the camel pose), and Gomukhasana (The cow pose) are suggested by Mitchell for bronchial congestion, and Balasana (the child's pose) with extended arms at the front and heading towards Bhujangasana (Cobra Pose) helps to open up the chest and inhibit pneumonia. However, if somehow you catch flu, it is better not to practice yoga since the condition requires complete rest. According to book Yoga for Health and Healing: From the teachings of Yogi Bhajan (1995), the Sukhasana (Easy Pose) with hands resting on the knees, thumb, and touching in Gyan (mudra) the index finger and breathing for a minimum over a U-shaped tongue.

The nasal and bronchial passages get blocked directly, and preventive actions can be taken to focus on these parts of the body. The yoga custom also recommends that less energy and poor digestion results in creating phlegm and mucus that travels in the lungs. This theory suggested that toxins build-up due to improper digestion turn into various diseases all over the body. Yoga poses helps to mildly twist, press, or extend the stomach that assists in various digestive complications.

The Power of Pranayama

As Asanas work like the foundation stone for the prevention of infection, the benefits of yoga do not just cease here. While bronchial passage gets attacked in the cold and flu symptoms, working on the lungs and making the most out of breathing aptitude through pranayama would help in building resistance against microbes. In the book, Yoda for Wellness (Penguin, 1999), Kraftsow explains that these lung infections like cold and flu, asthma, allergies, and other chronic bronchial problems are directly associated with a weakened immune system, because of irregular and improper breathing habits. Yoga practitioners emphasize on breathing exercises and training. Swift abdominal breathing and sectional breathing (Kapalbhati) advise that alternate-nostril breathing and nasal rinse enhances sinus resistance. A recent study from a Penn State University also supports this study after experimenting with it.

It is evident from the current situation of developing pandemics worldwide to build stress and anxiety from the social media and news world. Necessary precautions and recommended helpful at the first go along with the calmness of mind. Meditation proves to help reduce infection attacks by extracting stress from the body and mind. Much research demonstrates that just 20 minutes of meditation in a day boosts up endorphins in our body, decreases the levels of cortisol, and nurtures positivity of mind and body, promoting better health conditions.

So when should one begin a yoga program that helps in boosting immunity? Whatever your present yoga practice consists of, it is already working on your immunity and resistance strengthening. If you require taking extra footsteps for infection control, Richard Rosen, a YJ instructor and practitioner at Piedmont Yoga Studio in Oakland, California, advises forward and backbends along with twists provide support in boosting the immune system. Practicing the series daily, especially in winters, gives a better chance of staying healthy in cold seasons. If you perform to combat illness, these poses will provide the perfect rest and recuperation one needs to get better.

CHAPTER 10

IMMUNOTHERAPY AND ITS ROLE IN BOOSTING IMMUNE SYSTEM

So, we now know that our immune system is very adaptive and learns from its environment and its past experiences. But, what if you want to train your immune system to encounter problems they cannot in the state they are now. Yes, there are vaccines, but there are still some diseases that vaccines cannot cure like cancer and allergies. These diseases are caused by the immune system if they do not work correctly. Cancer is caused by a lack of awareness of the immune system, and allergies are caused by the immune system's over-sensitivity to a non-harmful substance. These are untreatable conditions but, with the development in science and immunology, we have found a way to train our excellent support staff to find the hidden culprit or to get over their sensitivity.

Immunotherapy trains our immune system on how to react to different substances and which cells are harmful and how to detect them. With time, scientists have developed two different types of immunotherapy. One is for allergies, and the other one is for cancer, let's begin with the one that is easier to understand.

Allergen Immunotherapy: As the name indicates, this type of immunotherapy works for maintaining allergies. The allergen immunotherapy works as exposure therapy, in which your body is exposed to the substance it is sensitive. Overtime body learns that it is not harmful, eliminating your allergy. If the allergy doesn't go at least, the deadly and life-threatening symptoms vanish, meaning that you can eat crab and peanuts. In the process of getting immunity from your allergies, it proceeds in two different methods. The subcutaneous route is in which you need to get injections every day. The duration depends upon your allergy. The dose contains a little bit of allergen in it that is injected in your body; the amount of allergen is increased day by day. The second method is a sublingual route in which a tablet or a drop of liquid is placed under the tongue. The method used for your symptoms depends upon the severity and the responsibility of the patient.

Cancer immunotherapy: Cancer immunotherapy is a procedure used in the treatment of patients with cancer while using immune system components. This statement looks like it came from a sci-fi movie, but it is being practiced to cure a lot of cancers. To cure cancer, we need to train our immune system like a beast, because malignancy can grow even if a single trace of it remains. To cure cancer, we use three types of immunotherapy.

- Non-specific immune stimulation

- T-Cell Transfer Therapy

- Immune Checkpoint Inhibitors

Let us start our discussion with non-specific immune stimulation. It is a type of immunotherapy in which the immune system is stimulated in general; no specific type of immune cell is aggravated. It is done by giving appropriate drugs and hormones to increase the production and activity of the immune cells. It is done to remove small cancers or to remove the trace of cancers after surgery. For example, if a person's bladder tumor is removed, the area is treated with a substance called BCG or bacille Calmette-Guerin, a vaccine for TB or tuberculosis. Surprisingly the vaccine increases the immune response, which results in proper removal of the traces of cancer that might have left during the surgery. It is a simple technique and works great for small cancers and tumors, but for more vicious cancers, we need to mutate our immune cells to get optimum results.

It is where T-Cell therapy comes in. In this type of treatment, your t-cells are trained and mutated to kill off the cancer cells. T-cells from your body are removed and then changes in the laboratory according to the patient's cancer cells. In the process, it is trained to identify cancerous cells lingering in your body undetected. Once the T-cells know which cells to target, they are replicated in a unique environment, so they stay healthy and strong. After they have reproduced in a substantial amount are allowed to enter our body through the drip. They show their training pretty conclusively in our bodies, but sometimes it does not work. It is because cancer cells are manipulative and wise, like any other traitor. They force the T-cells to go inactive and hide their receptors. It helps them to survive without any damage.

To counteract this, the third type of immunotherapy is taken under consideration Immune Checkpoint Inhibitors. Immune checkpoints on cell surfaces help control the immune response. Typically immune checkpoints hold T cells inactive until they are required, which is in an "off" state. It prevents T-cells from destroying healthy cells. Cancer cells may use certain checkpoints to turn off T cells. It avoids the destruction of the cancer cells. Immune checkpoint inhibitors are drugs blocking checkpoints. It frees the T-cells from attacking cancerous cells. All three types of immunotherapy are effective ways to treat cancer, but they do not work for every patient and can cause severe side effects. National Cancer Institute-backed researchers are working on learning more about how the immune system works to combat cancer. By researching this in both cases, researchers will know how to develop immunotherapy.

Immunotherapy is a vast subject that has helped to treat a lot of patients, but with a success rate of 20%, the chances are pretty slim but worth trying. Immunotherapy still has to cover a long journey to be a successful treatment for cancers. As far as immunotherapy for allergies is concerned, it is beneficial, but because every human body has a different type of immune response, results vary slightly. Immunotherapy is a revolutionary concept, and maybe in the future, we can use it to defeat some of the deadliest diseases as well, or perhaps it can be used to regrow an amputated leg or an arm or finger at least. Immunotherapy has helped many people, and it can change the way our immune system operates.

Benefits of a boosted Immune system

A robust immune response is one of the significant benefits for humans, and many steps can be taken by individuals to help strengthen their immune systems to help fight infections and reduce the risk of highly contagious diseases. When we usually hear a robust immune system, we get an image of a person who is hard to get sick. Which is true, but we undermine the other benefits that come with boosted or healthy immune system. A hearty immune system, especially in old age, i.e., the seventies, will make you not only look like but feel like you still feel like you are in your early twenties. A robust immune system offers a higher age expectancy and way fewer chances of getting cancer. If you are allergic to something, boosting your immune system and working out daily might help get rid of it.

The best is that you have a high chance of surviving a pandemic or an epidemic even when you are in your old age. A boosted immune system can make your logical perception better because of fewer distractions in your body. Your brain can think and perform better, but more studies are required to back this info. All the tips mentioned will help you get a lifestyle that you want. Even if you are in your prime and think that there is nothing that you can do, then you so wrong. Being healthy doesn't depend on your age and time; it depends upon your determination and motivation.

Implementing all of these tips is not easy in your daily life, but thinking that you can never do that and don't even bother to start implementing these is not helpful at all. All you need is a start, and you can catch up with the pace.

Start small and build up your way. You don't need fancy supplements to have a healthy immune system and an immune response. Now you know a lot about the immune system, and from this data, you can evaluate whether which foodstuffs and what method should be the best for you. If your immune system is not in good condition, you will look old and might feel lazy and tired all the time. To overcome these symptoms, you should have a routine that offers a healthy immune system with a proper lifestyle.

You don't have to be too strict, but should be regular. Evaluate yourself and find the reason of your cold symptoms you have to suffer now and then. Having a more robust immune system, we go from a sterilization system to where bacterial colonization is a norm. A little determination and some knowledge can make a difference of day and night.

That's the end of this great little book. Like my Facebook page, Follow me on Twitter and visit website to share about your health and discussion.

https://www.facebook.com/HealthyFitCareOfficial

https://twitter.com/hfc__official

https://healthyfitcare.com

Stay Blessed and Safe

Aadil A. Abbasi